HARRY AND HIS BIG LITTLE FAMILY

Written and Illustrated By:
TeArra M. Boone

This is Harry Bonds with his mom and dad Frank and Kate. They are all very big. They love to eat. That is what they live for.

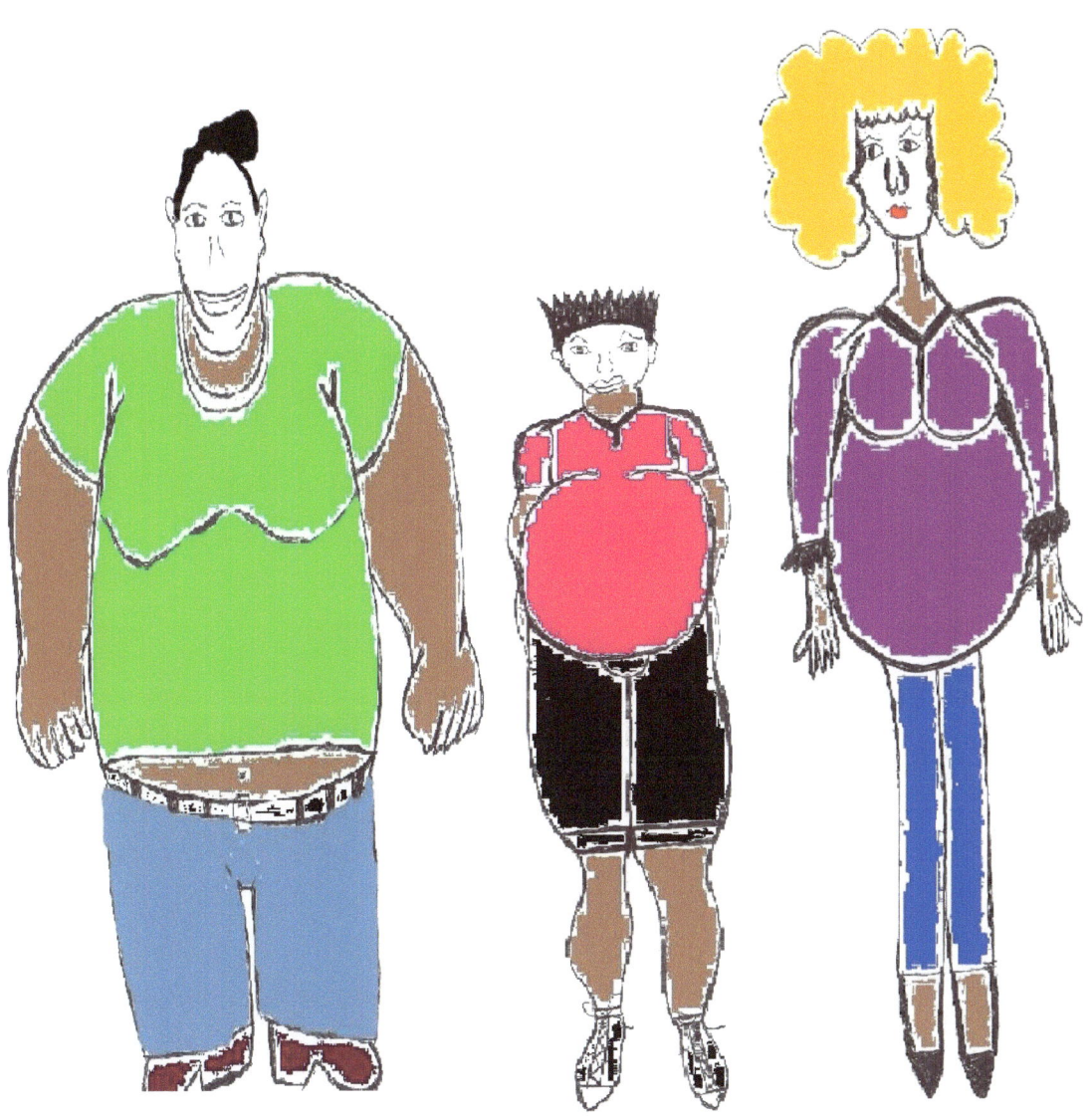

At school Harry is teased because of his fat.

"Hey Harry," said one kid, "Why do you have so many belly's?"

"JELLY ROLL," said another kid.

"You're so fat you could pretend you're a cow and live on a farm," said another.

They would just not leave poor Harry alone.

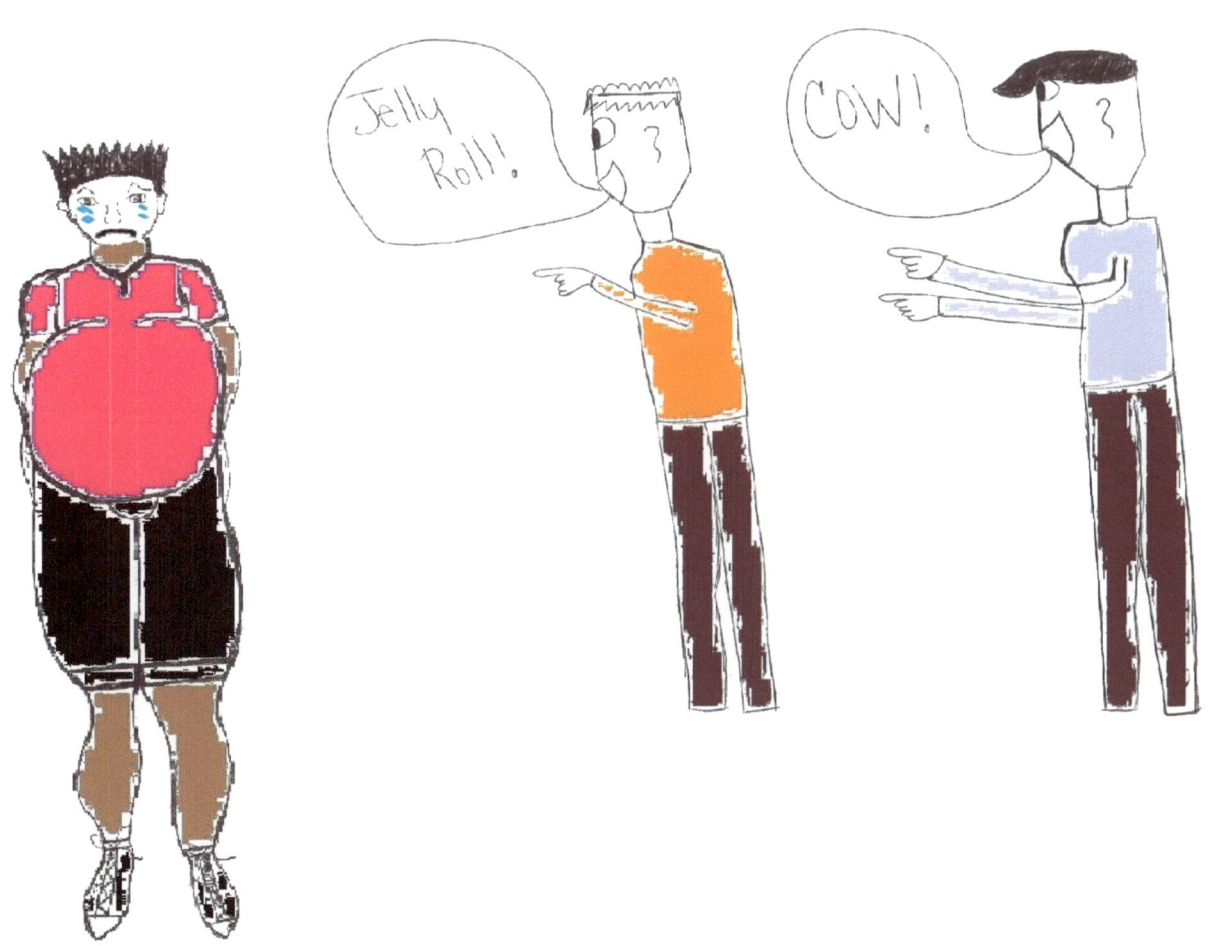

When Harry went home he cried his eyes out to his mommy. "Why are they so mean? Why am I so fat?," Harry said.

Harry's mom wiped his tears and told him to take a nap so that he could calm down.

While Harry was sleeping he had a dream that he was exercising and said no to all the junk food in the world.
He became very healthy and was never called fat again by anyone.

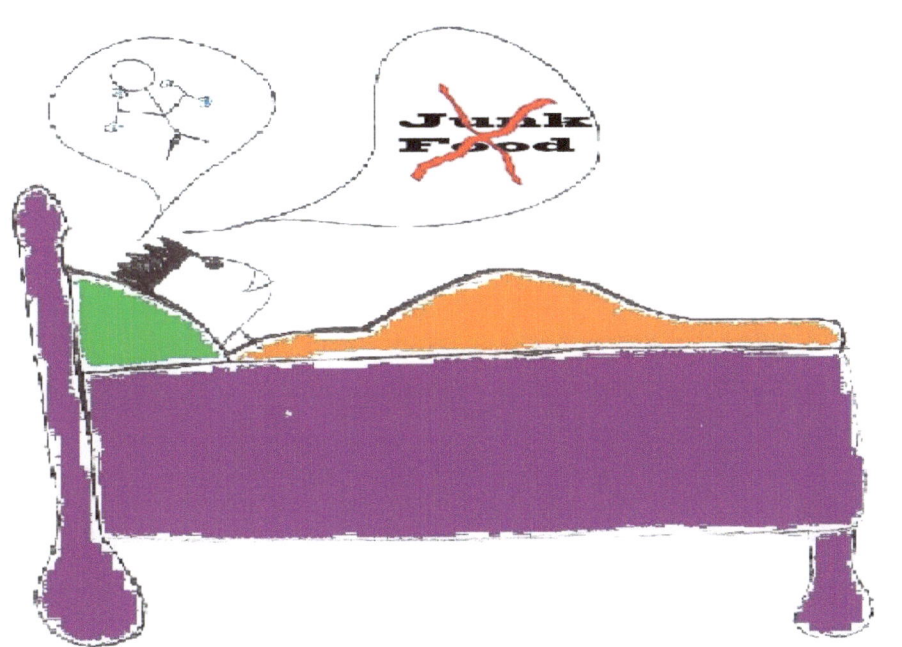

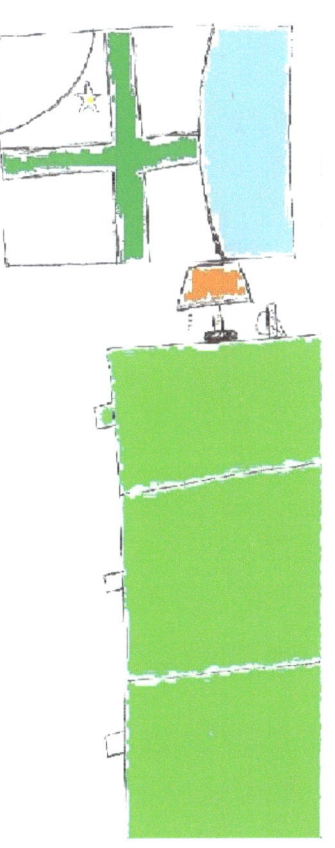

Excited because of his dream, Harry ran downstairs to his mother and told her that he wanted to be a healthy kid and never ever wanted to see or eat anymore candy, popcorn, chips, or corn dogs.

He wanted only fruit and vegetables.

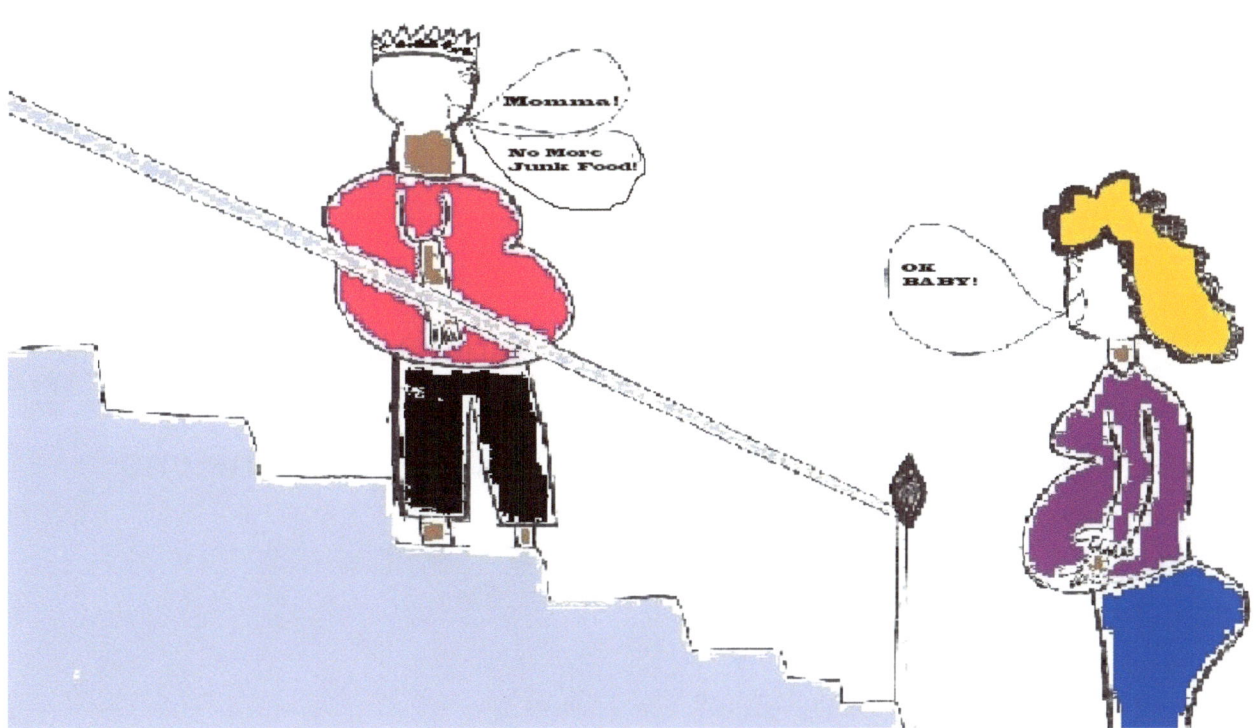

That same night, before dinner, Harry began to exercise in his room.

He did sit-ups, push-ups, and jumping jacks. The jumping jacks did not work out that well because when he did them he shook the entire house, but in the end he was proud.

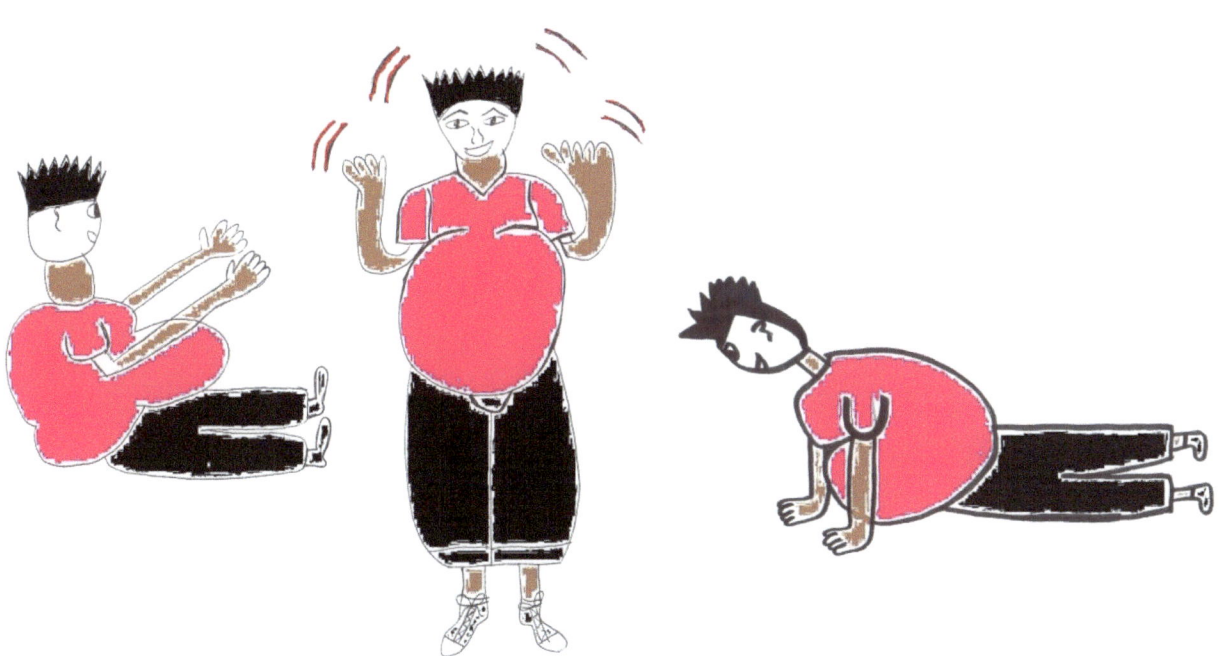

After the weekend was over, it was back to school for Harry. He was excited to go because it was the last day of school for Summer.

Harry was surprised because no one teased him that day. He knew he was getting healthy after all. After the day was over, Harry went home with a smile on his face.

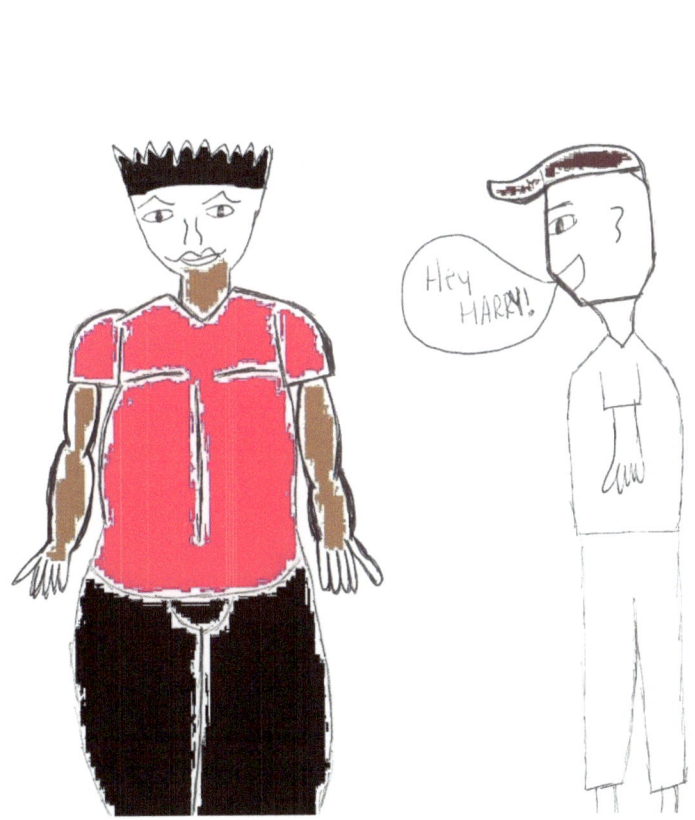
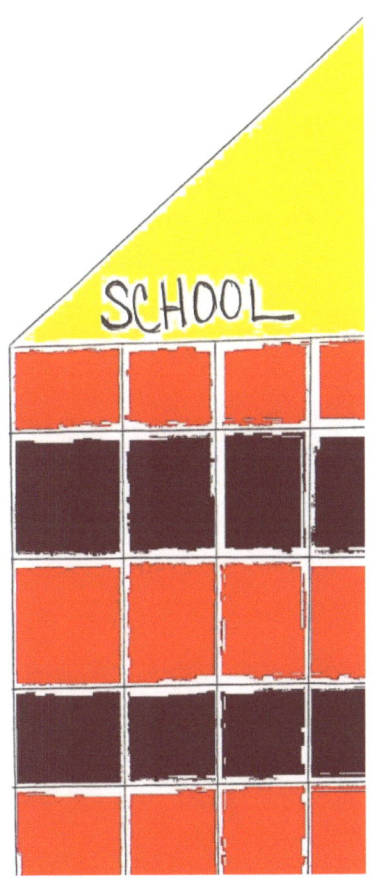

Later after his dinner of corn, turkey, and some more broccoli, Harry decided to do some exercising.

Then he watched some television.

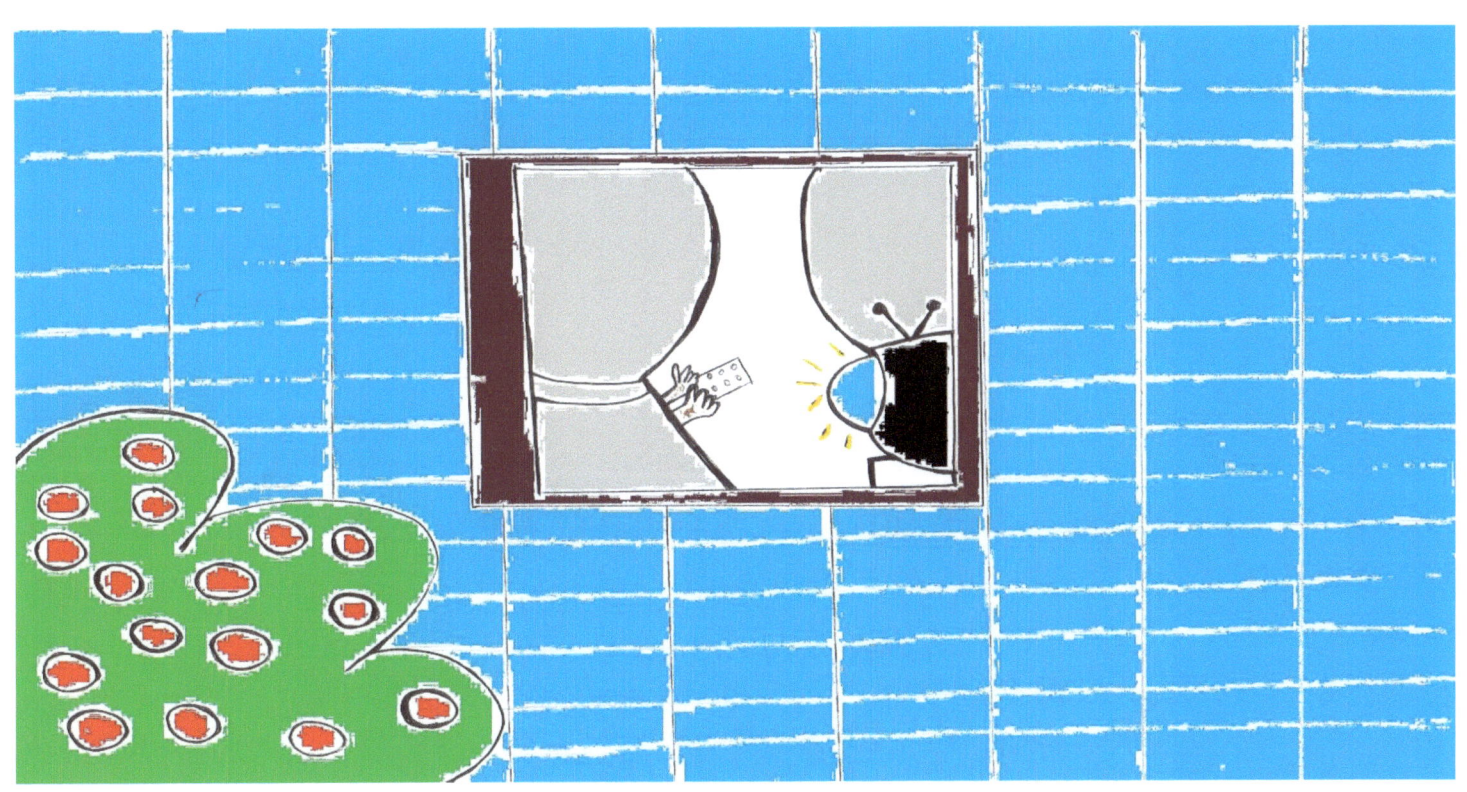

A commercial came on about a camp just for people that wanted to exercise. Harry could not believe that there was such a thing.

He begged for his mom's permission to go. She agreed and Harry rushed up the steps to pack his things since he was leaving in two days.

The next day Harry and his family went to a restaurant and his parents decided to let him have a piece of chocolate cake since he did so well with his exercising. He really enjoyed it.

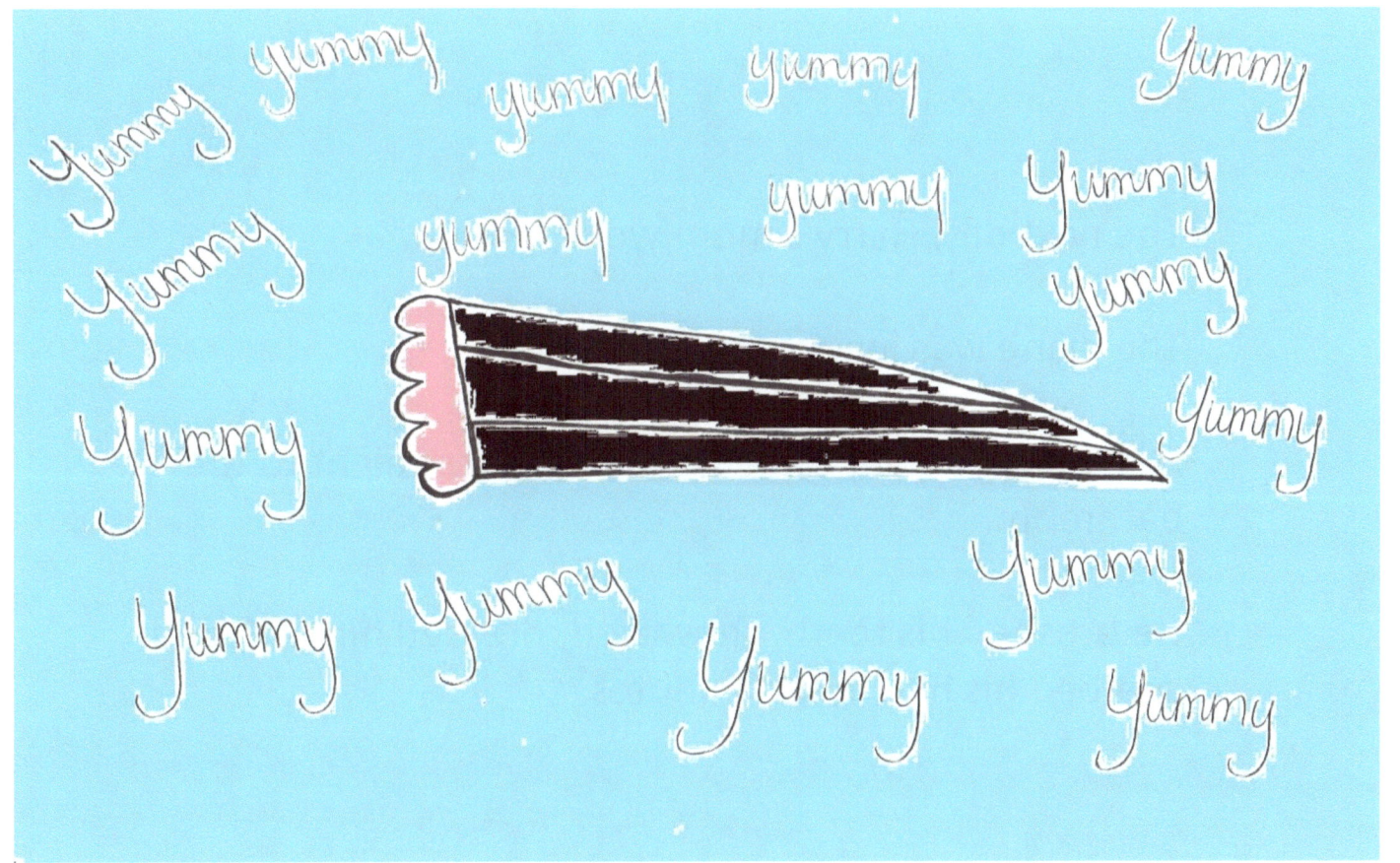

When he arrived home Harry exercised, then went straight to bed.

The next day, Harry's mom woke him up.

The plane was leaving in two hours.

Harry jumped out of bed and headed straight to the bathroom.

He brushed his teeth, showered, dressed himself, and combed his hair in ten minutes.

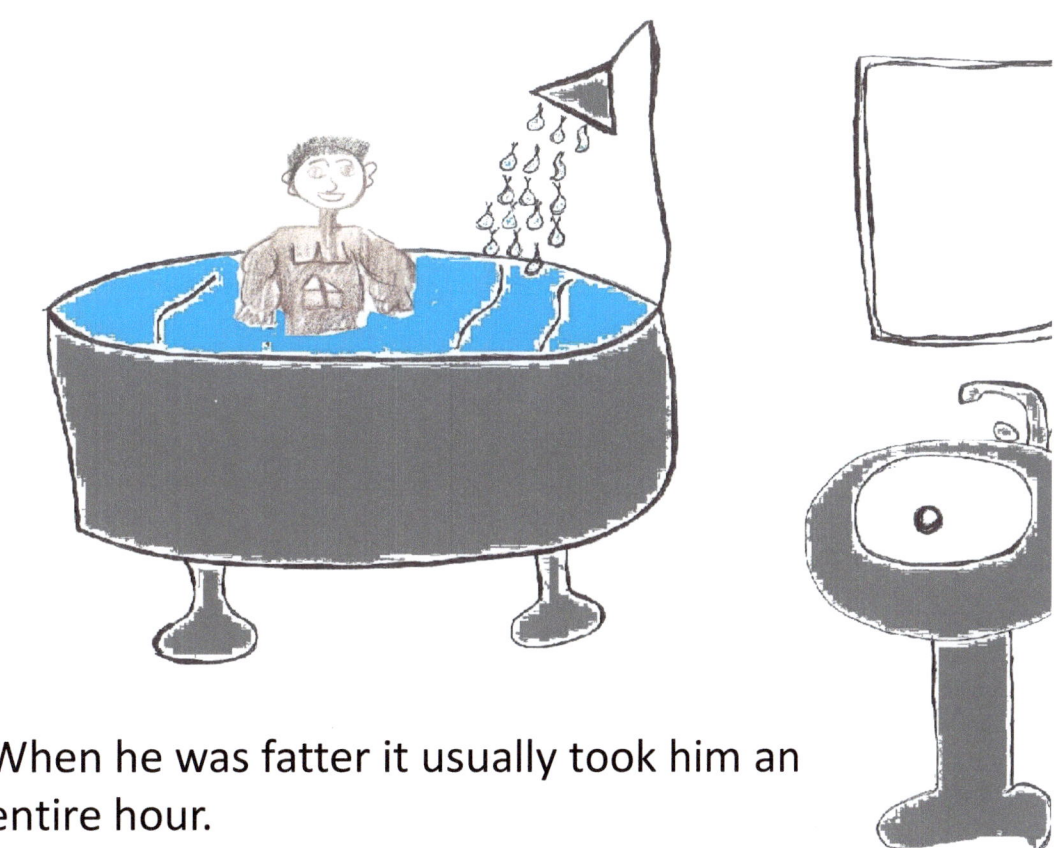

When he was fatter it usually took him an entire hour.

The exercising camp lasted for three fast months with many of the activities that Harry played before.

They played sports that the boys never let Harry play at school.

Harry was having a blast and became much more healthier, but it was time to go home.

Harry said his goodbyes to his friends and headed for the airport. "Goodbye Jordan, Lucy, Howard, Roger, Betty, and Lulu. I'll miss you a lot."

His mom and dad came to get him from the airport, but he could hardly recognize them. They became healthy too.

Two days after arriving home, Harry had to go back to school.

He could not wait to show off his healthiness.

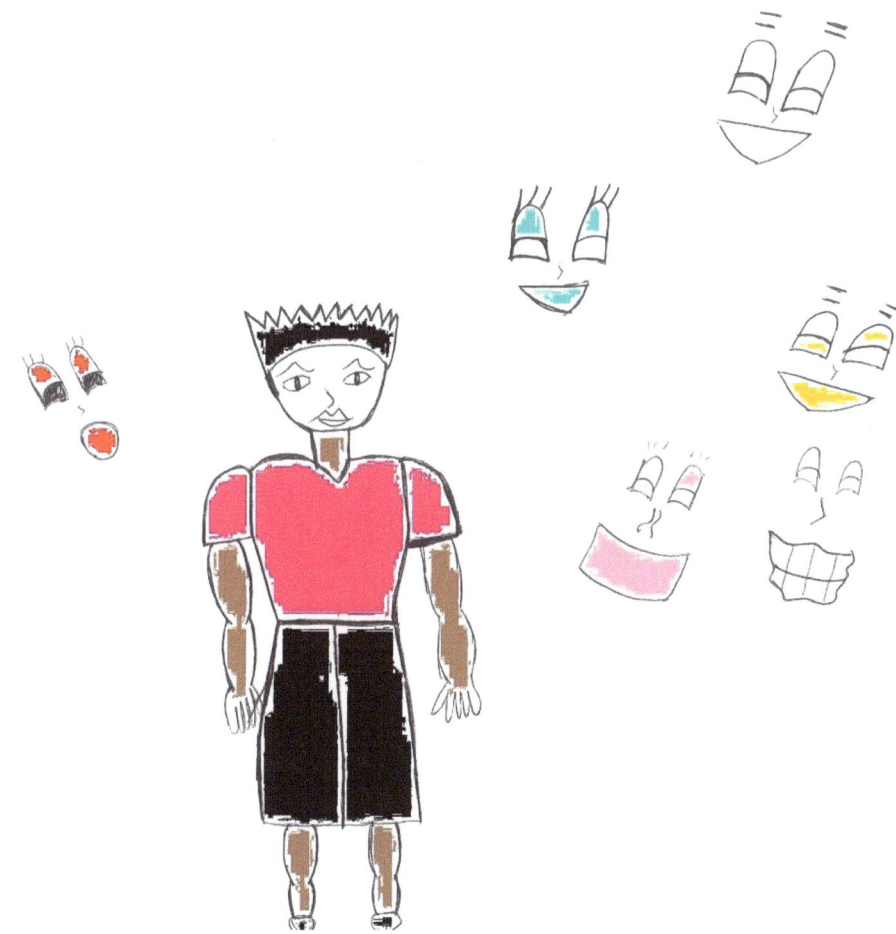

Everyone was very shocked to see how much Harry had changed.

They let him play football, basketball, soccer, and now they were not even afraid to wrestle him anymore.

Even his crush Jada gave him a kiss.

He couldn't believe it. He loved being healthy even more.

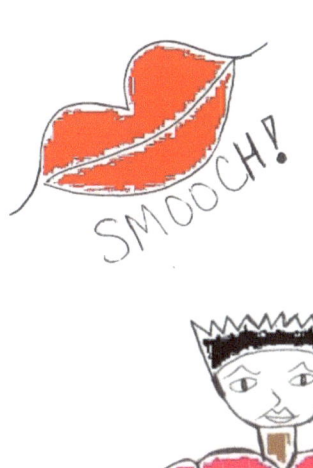

SMOOCH!

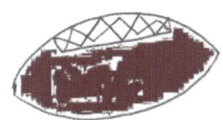

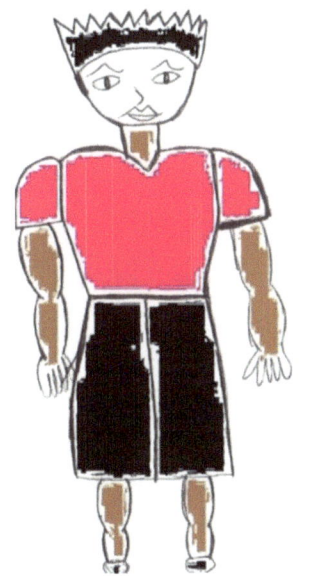

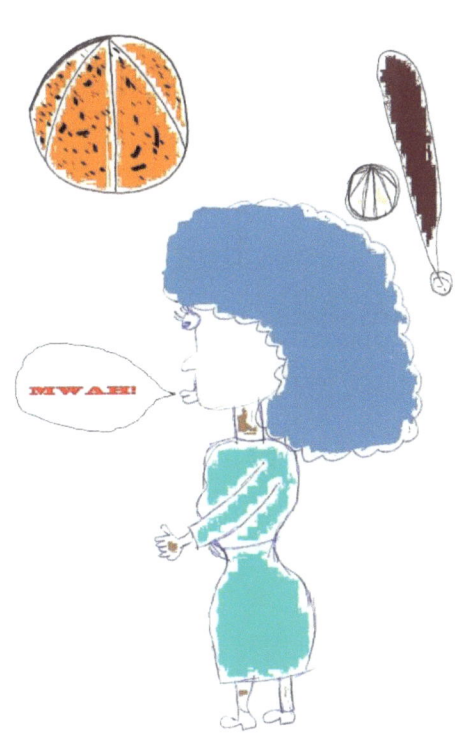

MWAH!

Harry exercised everyday now and even taught his friends how to.

He learned that being healthy is the best thing and is proud that he chose to be healthy.

If Harry can be healthy, you can too!

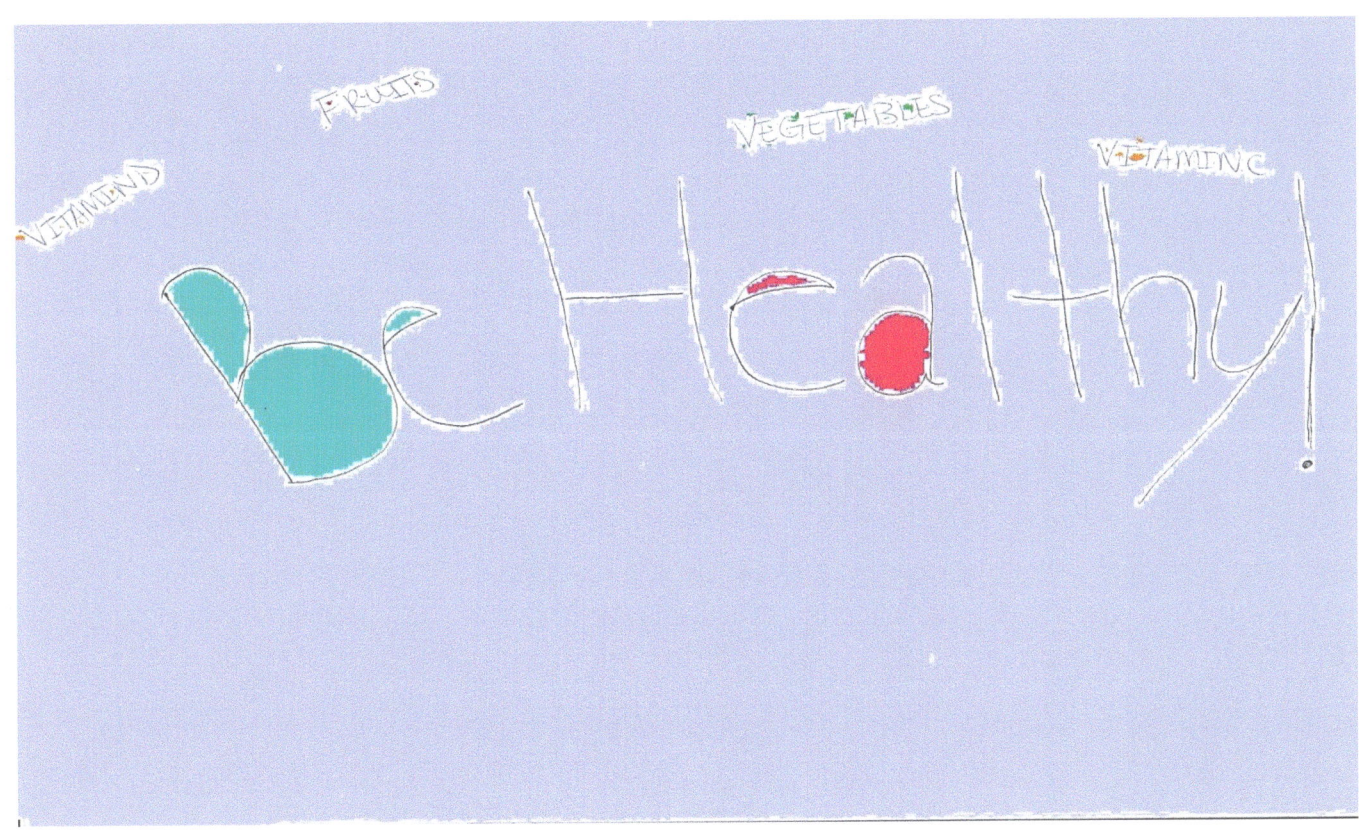